I0424068

Fruit Infused Water

77 Refreshing Vitamin Fruit Infusion Water Recipes For A Healthier You

AMELIA LONG

ISBN-13:978-1515265887

ISBN-10:1515265889

DEDICATION

To God, for the wonderful gift of nature

TABLE OF CONTENT

Other Books by Amelia Long

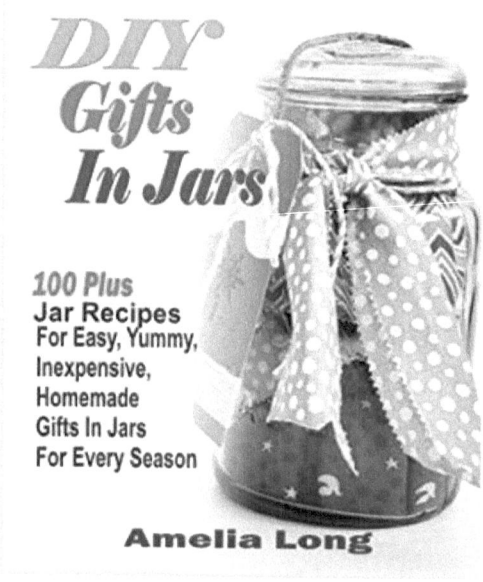

DIY Gifts In Jars:100 Plus Jar Recipes For Easy, Yummy, Inexpensive, Homemade Gifts In Jars For Every Season

INTRODUCTION

The human body cannot function without water. Water cleanses the body, eliminates toxins, carries nutrients to the cells, provides a moist environment for tissues and beautifies the skin. According to the Institute of Medicine, a man needs about 13 cups (roughly3 liters) of total beverages daily while a woman requires about 9 cups (2.2 liters) of total beverages daily. To many people, drinking plain old boring water is a chore that they strive to carry out. However, with fruit infused waters, its rich subtle flavor ensure you can never get tired of drinking it. It tastes great. It is gentle, refreshing and keeps you hydrated.

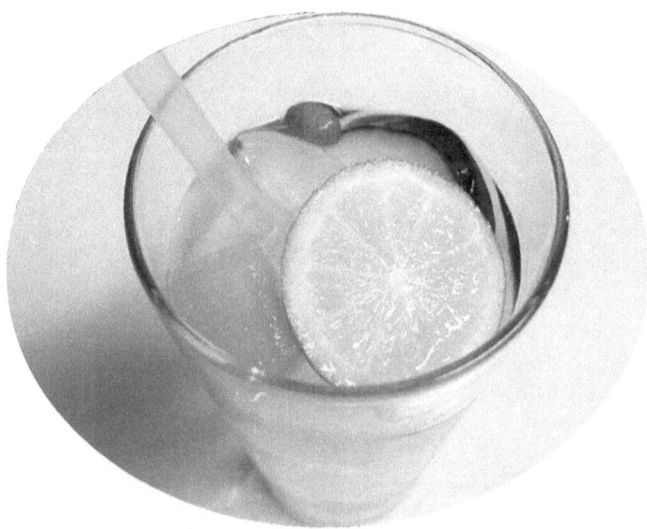

Infused waters are pleasantly easy to make and come with a burst of color and a slight hint of fresh flavor. The superb thing about them is that they are all natural. The fruits and herbs that grow right outside your garden is all it takes to make them. They are wonderfully refreshing during summer. They are simple to make and very affordable. You can also have fun making them as you try all sorts of combinations. You can choose your preferred combination and mix the fruits as you like. There is really no end to what you can make. Even if you drink up the water within the first day, just add more filtered water and infuse again to get a second use and benefit out of the fruits and herbs.

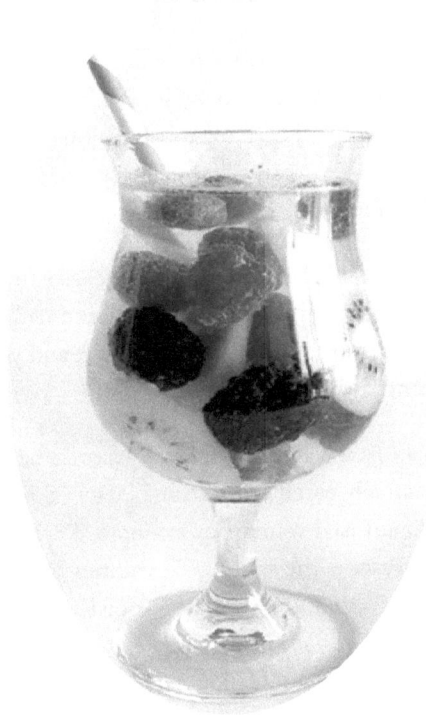

Ditch the juice for fruit infused water. Juice is definitely
not the answer. A better way to quench your thirst is by
taking herbs and fruits infused waters. They help to
improve the flavor while providing the nutritional value
that is needed. All it takes is to simply let fruits and herbs
sit in water for a couple of hours and there! You have your
alternative to plain 'ole boring water and potential harmful
juice. They are also delicious as well.

A Few Benefits Of Fruits Infused Water

Hydration— fruit infused water keeps you hydrated. We all know that lack of water leads to dehydration but by drinking infused water and carrying a batch along with you all day, it becomes easier to stay hydrated especially when the weather is blazing hot.

Good Health — fruit infused water makes it easier for you to stay healthy. You have healthier skin, hair and nails. Your energy is increased, you are mentally alert and your focus and concentration is heightened.

Calories— fruit infused waters have fewer calories because the fruit is not actually eaten but remains intact. You need less fruit to make infused water. For example, 3 orange slices in infused water is the same as 31 calories or even less. This is good for you. It also makes it easier to achieve weight loss.

Flavor— fruit rinds infused in water brings out the flavor even after only 15 minutes of infusion. The taste is tangy and bright as a result.

Appearance— The infused water looks good. With its pleasing appearance, you look forward to drinking it over and over again.

Preparation— it is easy to prepare. Just take a glance at what is available and improvise.

Less consumption of sugar-based drinks— say goodbye to sugar- based drinks. Who needs them when you can enjoy optimum health benefits from delicious and soothingly refreshing fruit and herbs infused water.

STRAWBERRY INFUSED WATER RECIPES

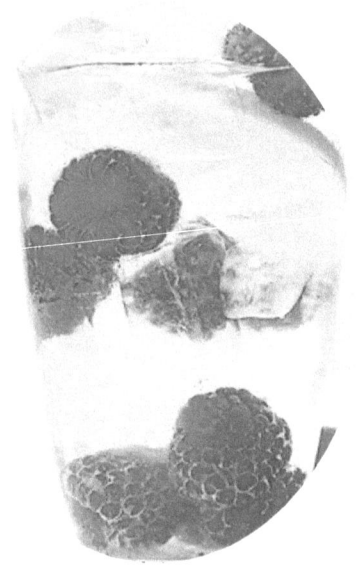

Strawberry, Basil and Lemon Water

Ingredients

2 tablespoons fresh lemon juice

5 strawberries, sliced

6 fresh basil leaves

1 tablespoon raw honey

3/4 cups of water

1 pinch salt

Directions

1. Combine the lemon juice, basil, strawberries and raw honey in a large glass. Mix together until the honey dissolves.

2. Add ice cubes and water, stir and keep until chilled.

3. Next, strain the mixture into a glass containing ice cubes.

No-Rind Strawberry Lemon Water

This is a great recipe to try if you have strawberries that are going bad in your refrigerator. The berries will be infused in chilled water and this helps to prolong its shelf life. Lemon rinds must be removed so it does not overpower the strawberries' flavor.

Ingredients

1 lemon with rind removed, slice

5 strawberries

Directions

1. Combine in a pitcher. Add purified water and refrigerate for at least 4 hours.

2. This recipe is for an 80 oz Water Pitcher.

Strawberry And Lime Water

Ingredients

8 large strawberries, thinly sliced

1 cucumber, thinly sliced

2 limes, juiced

Directions

1. Add together all the ingredients in a pitcher.

2. Add cold water, cover, and store in the refrigerator overnight.

Strawberry & Pineapple Water

Ingredients

1 cup of strawberries (sliced)

1 cored pineapple

Ice and Water

Directions

1. Add the pineapple and strawberries in a large pitcher.

2. Fill with water and refrigerate for 2 to 4 hours.

Strawberry & Basil

Ingredients

10 strawberries, sliced thinly

3 basil leaves, torn and muddled

2 quarts water

Directions

1. Pour water over the strawberries and basil. Refrigerate 2 hours.

2. Serve over ice, garnished with 1 sprig of basil.

Strawberry Infused Water

Ingredients

8 fresh cucumber slices

4 sliced strawberries

½ gallon water

Directions

1. Add the strawberries and cucumber in a large pitcher and fill with water.

2. Refrigerate about 4 hours. Serve in ice-filled glasses.

Berries Fusion

Ingredients

2 cups blueberries, slightly muddled

10 strawberries, thinly sliced

2 quarts water

Directions

1. Add the blueberries and strawberries to a pitcher.

2. Fill with water and refrigerate for 4 hours.

Strawberry& Lemon Fusion

Ingredients

15 fresh strawberries, finely sliced

1 sliced lemon (with rind on)

1/2 gallon water

Directions

1. Add all together in a glass jar.

2. Let it sit refrigerate 4 hours or overnight. Enjoy!

Strawberry, Cucumber, Lime and Mint Medley

Ingredients

1 cup sliced cucumbers

1 cup sliced strawberries

1/4 cup fresh mint leaves

2 limes, sliced

Water

Ice cubes

Directions

1. Add the cucumbers, strawberries, mint leaves and lime slices to a 1/2 gallon jar.

2. Add the ice cubes and then fill the jar with water.

3. Let it chill for about 10 minutes and enjoy.

4. Garnish with a strawberry slice.

CITRUS INFUSED WATER RECIPES

Kumquats, Orange & Nasturtium Infusion
Ingredients

1 organic orange, sliced

1 1/2cup of kumquats, sliced &seeded

1 handful nasturtium flowers

2 quarts water

Directions:

1. Combine them all in a pitcher.

2. Cover and let it chill for 1 hour. Serve with ice cubes

Grapefruit & Raspberry
Ingredients

1grapefruit, thinly sliced

½ cup fresh raspberries

Directions

1. Add all to water, mixing well.

2. Refrigerate 4-7 hours and enjoy!

Citrus Mix

Ingredients

1 lime, sliced thinly

1 orange, sliced thinly

1/2 of a lemon, thinly sliced

2 quarts of water

Directions

1. Add the lime, orange and lemon to the water Refrigerate for at least 4 hours.

2. Serve over ice, garnished with 1 sprig of basil.

Citrus & Coriander Blend

Ingredients

1 large lemon, sliced

1 large orange, sliced

1 large lime, sliced

1/4 cup of cilantro leaves

Directions

1. Pour water over the citrus fruits and cilantro. Let it chill for 2 hours.

2. Serve over ice, garnished with a sprig of cilantro and an orange slice.

Lemon& Cucumber Waters

Ingredients

12 thinly sliced cucumber

4 thinly sliced lemon

6 cups of still spring or mineral water, chilled

Directions

1. Combine cucumber, lemon and water in a 2-2 ½ quart pitcher.

2. Cover and chill 2 to 8 hours. Add ice cubes and serve immediately.

Cherry Lime

Ingredients

2 cups fresh cherries

1 fresh lime, sliced thinly

Directions

1. Add cherries and lime to a glass jar (gallon size)

2. Add water to fill, mix and refrigerate.

Spicy Tangerine

Ingredients:

4 tangerines sliced

3 sprigs thyme

3 sprigs fennel

2 quarts water

Directions:

1. Add all together in a 2 quarts pitcher.

2. Let it infuse for 2 to 4 hours in the fridge.

Herby Lime

Ingredients

1 lime, sliced

2 fresh basil leaves

4-6 fresh peppermint leaves

1/2 gallon water

Directions

1. Add ingredients to a pitcher.

2. Cover, and chill for about 30 minutes.

3. Finally, strain, add ice, pour into glasses and serve.

Cucumber, Mint And Lemon Infused Water

Ingredients

1 lemon, slice into rounds

1 large cucumber, slice into rounds

Water

1 handful mint leaves

1 handful ice (optional)

Directions

1. Place the mint into a1½ quart container and muddle gently to release flavor.

2. Add cucumber, lemon to container and then fill it with ice and water.

3. Stir and refrigerate 4 hours or overnight.

Citrus Cucumber Medley

Ingredients

1 large cucumber, sliced

1 large lime, sliced

1 large lemon, sliced

1 large orange, sliced

½ gallon of water

Directions

1. Place all the ingredients in a glass pitcher. Add the water.

2. Let it infuse for 2 hours. Serve over ice.

Orange Mint Water

Ingredients

3 large oranges, sliced

10 mint leaves

½ gallon of water

Directions

1. Place mint and orange in a pitcher and the add water. Infuse 2 hours in the refrigerator.

2. Next, pour over ice and serve garnished with a sprig of mint and an orange slice.

Grape Orange Blend

Ingredients

1 orange, thinly sliced

2 cups grapes, sliced in half

Directions

1. Add all to ½ gallon glass jar

2. Refrigerate overnight.

Lemon Lavender Medley

Ingredients

1/4 cup fresh lavender

3 large lemons, thickly sliced

½ gallon of water

Directions

1. Pour the ½ gallon water over the lavender and lemons.

2. Refrigerate 2 hours and serve over ice. Garnish with 1 sprig of lavender.

Orange & Vanilla Infusion
Ingredients

1 orange, sliced

2 liters filtered water

1/2 teaspoon of vanilla extract, or1 vanilla bean, scraped

Directions:

1. Combine all the ingredients in a large pitcher.

2. Mix thoroughly and refrigerate.

3. This makes 2 liters

Orange Blueberry
Ingredients

6 cups of ice water

2 mandarin oranges (cut into wedges)

1 handful blueberries

Directions

1. Combine all the ingredients in a pitcher and refrigerate 2 to 24 hours.

2. Alternatively, squeeze in the juice of a mandarin orange and mix the blueberries to intensify the flavor.

FRUIT INFUSED WATER RECIPES WITH MINT

Cucumber Mint

Ingredients

1 cucumber, thinly sliced

8 fresh mint leaves

½ gallon water

Directions

1. Add cucumber, water and mint leaves to 1/2 gallon glass jar.

2. Stir gently, refrigerate overnight or at least for 4 hours.

Cherry Minty

Ingredients

1 sprig of mint

1 Key lime, thinly sliced

6 pitted cherries cut in1/2

Directions

1. Combine and let it steep for 30 minutes.

2. Chill or serve it over ice.

Blueberry/ Mint Infused Waters

Ingredients

2 cups of blueberries

2 sprigs mint, muddled

2 quarts water

Directions

1. Place the muddled mint, blueberries and water in a container.

2. Stir and refrigerate 4 hours or overnight.

Pineapple Mint Medley

Ingredients

2 sprigs mint

4 pineapple slices

1 quart water and ice

Directions

For a stronger flavor, chill or serve immediately for light refreshment.

Spicy Cucumber Mint Dill Infused Water

This herb and cucumber mixture is light and refreshing and pairs wonderfully well with sandwiches.

Ingredients

2/3 cucumber, with peel cut off

6-8 fresh mint leaves, torn

3 sprigs fresh dill

Directions

1. Layer 3 to 4 slices of cucumber, 1 sprig of dill and 2 torn mint leaves in a 93-oz pitcher. Repeat layering.

2. Infuse overnight or for about 6 hours for optimum flavor.

Minty Strawberries

Ingredients

16 medium sized Strawberries (sliced thin)

1 quart water and ice

8 sprigs of mint

Directions

1. Combine. Leave for 30 minutes and then serve.

Minty Watermelon Delight

Ingredients

1 watermelon, medium-sized& chopped

2 tbsp mint leaves

Chaat masala to taste (optional)

Ice cubes

Black salt to taste

Directions

1. Add the mint leaves and watermelon in a blender and puree.

2. Pour into a glass of ice cubes. Garnish with black salt and chaat masala, if using.

Honeydew Mint Water

Ingredients

1 lime, sliced

4 sprigs of mint

2 or 3 slices of ripe honeydew melon

½ gallon water

Directions

1. Add mint sprigs, melon slices and lime slices to a large pitcher. Add water to pitcher.

2. Refrigerate for 2 to 4 hours. Serve drink in ice-filled glasses.

FRUIT INFUSED WATER WITH TEA RECIPES

Green Tea/ Mango Infused Water

Ingredients:

1 green tea bag

1 cup mango, pureed & ripe

1 tablespoon of honey

1 quart water

Directions:

1. Boil the water and add the tea bags to the boiled water. Let it steep 5 minutes.

2. Take out the tea bags and then pour the tea water into a jar.

3. Add the honey and mango puree. Refrigerate at least 2 hours.

4. Strain and then serve.

Lemon Strawberry Iced Tea

Ingredients

2 lemons, sliced

8-10 large strawberries, sliced

1 strawberry lemonade Tea

2 quarts of water

Directions:

1. Boil the water. Place the tea in it and let it steep for 2 to 3 minutes. (only a little tea flavor is needed).

2. Pour the tea water into a jar. Add the sliced lemons and strawberries.

3. Fill the jar with water and then place in the fridge for 2-4 hours.

4. Serve over ice.

Strawberry Fruit Infusion

Ingredients

1 Cup of Strawberries Sliced

5 Small Bags Lipton Tea

10 Cups of Water

2 trays of ice

½-3/4 Cup White Sugar

Directions

1. Place the tea bags and water in a stock pot and bring just to a boil. Add the sugar and stir and bring to a boil.

2. Next, remove from heat, take out the tea bag and then add the strawberries.

3. Let it steep15- 20 minutes. Remove the strawberries.

4. Now add the ice to mixture and serve cold.

5. Garnish with strawberries. This serves 5.

Starfruit, Orange And Hibiscus Tea Medley

Ingredients:

5 slices of cored starfruit

1 orange, sliced

2 bags of hibiscus tea

2 quarts water

Directions:

1. Add together all ingredients.

2. Refrigerate overnight.

Blueberry Black Iced Tea Delight

Ingredients:

1 blueberry black tea

20 cubes watermelon

1 cup blueberries

3 peaches, sliced

2 quarts of water

Directions:

1. Boil the water and steep the tea in the boiled water for at least 3 minutes to release some flavor.

2. To a jar or pitcher, add the tea water and the rest of the ingredients.

3. Let it chill for at least four hours. Serve over ice.

FRUIT INFUSED WATER GENERAL RECIPES

Pink Rose Vanilla Infused Water

Ingredients:

1/4 cup of dried pink rose petals

1/2 large vanilla bean

3/4 cup of frozen or fresh raspberries

2 quarts water

Directions:

1. Slice the vanilla bean lengthwise and muddle the raspberries.

2. Add everything together in a jar.

3. Refrigerate overnight and strain the next day before drinking

Refreshing Blueberry Lavender

Ingredients

1/2 pint Blueberries

64 ounces Water

Lavender flowers, to taste

Directions

1. Add ingredients to a pitcher.

2. Cover, and chill for about 30 minutes.

3. Finally, strain, add ice, pour into glasses and serve. (This makes 8 servings).

Berry Rosemary Water

Ingredients

2 4–inch sprigs fresh rosemary, lightly bruised (to release extra flavor)

1 cup of fresh blueberries, lightly crushed

½ gallon of water

Directions

1. Add the rosemary sprigs and blueberries to a large pitcher. Fill with water.

2. Refrigerate about 4 hours and then serve in ice-filled glasses.

Melon Cucumber Water
Ingredients

1/4 honeydew melon, cubed

1 large cucumber, sliced

1/4 cantaloupe, cubed

½ gallon of water

Directions

1. Place cucumber and melon in a glass pitcher. Add water.

2. Refrigerate 2 hours and then serve over ice. Garnish with skewered melon balls on a swizzle stick

Frozen Fruits Delight
Ingredients

2 cups frozen grapes, apple chunks or berries

1 half-gallon of water

Directions

1. Add the frozen fruit to a pitcher and then pour water over it.

2. Refrigerate 30 minutes to 2 hours Stir to mix fruit flavor well and serve in glasses with ice cubes.

Cinnamon &Pear

Ingredients:

5 pears, sliced

2 cinnamon sticks

1 small lemon, sliced in half

2 quarts of water

Directions:

1. Place the sliced pears in a jar.

2. Squeeze half of the sliced lemon over the pear. Thinly slice the other half lemon left and throw into the jar.

3. Add cinnamon to it, fill with water and cover. Let it chill at least 2 hours to infuse. Serve over ice.

Watermelon and Basil

Ingredients

 2 cups seedless watermelon, cubed

10 to 12 basil leaves

½ gallon water

Directions

1. Pour water over the basil and melon. Refrigerate 2 hours.

2. Serve over ice, garnished with 1 sprig of basil.

Peach, Thyme and Blackberry Infused Water

Ingredients:

2 peaches

1 pint blackberries

2 sprigs of thyme

Water

4 cups ice

Directions:

1. Muddle the blackberries and peaches in a jar using a wooden spoon.

2. Add the water, thyme and ice.

Special Blueberry Blend

Ingredients

1/4 cup dried lavender

1/2 cup fresh blueberries

10 lemons

1/12 cups very hot water

3/4 -1 cup honey or raw sugar, to taste

2 tbsp water

Directions

1. Add the water and dried lavender to a teapot or bowl and let it steep for about 10 minutes.

2. Strain the water into a pitcher and then add the honey or sugar and stir until it dissolves.

3. Add ice to the mixture and let it cool for a while.

4. Juice the lemons, add it to the pitcher and then add cold water at the same time.

5. In a blender, puree the blueberries with 2 tablespoons water and then add to the lemonade, immediately.

6. Stir well and enjoy

Raspberry Basil
Ingredients

1 handful quartered raspberries

10-12 fresh basil leaves

1/2 gallon of water

Directions

1. Add all the ingredients together.

2. Stir gently, refrigerate overnight or at least for 4 hours.

Mango& Pineapple

Ingredients

1 mango, sliced thinly

1 cup pineapple

Directions

1. Add the mango to a 1/2 gallon glass jar. Add the pineapple and then add water.

2. Let it infuse in the fridge for at least 4 hours before serving.

Cilantro Infused Seltzer Water

Ingredients

2 or 3 stems organic cilantro

1 liter of seltzer water

Ice

Directions

1. Put the cilantro stems in a glass and add the ice.

2. Fill with seltzer water. Enjoy!

Lemon Thyme & Blackberry

Ingredients:

1 handful blackberries (frozen or fresh)

3 sprigs lemon thyme

2 quarts of water

Directions:

1. Place the lemon thyme and blackberries in a 2 quart jar.

2. Fill it with water and then chill for a few hours.

FRUIT INFUSED WATER FOR VARIOUS HEALTH BENEFITS

Anti-Bloating Remedy

Ingredients

2 sliced lemons

1/2 cucumber, sliced

1 fresh mint leaves

2 tsp chopped ginger root

3 qt. water

Directions

1. Add mint, ginger, cucumber, lemon and water to a pitcher.

2. Cover overnight. Serve hot or chilled.

Green Power-Health Waters

The cucumbers in this vegetable and herb infused water helps to reduce bloating, the jalapeño peppers increase your metabolism while the mint relieves headaches and aids digestion.

Ingredients

3/4 cucumber sliced

1 sprig mint leaves

1/2 jalapeño pepper, de-seeded

Directions

1. In a 32 oz Ball jar, combine all the ingredients and then cover it with cold water.

2. Let it chill infused for 4 to 24 hours for best flavors.

Immune Booster

Ingredients

1 cup cubed pineapple

1 cup strawberries, chopped

2 peeled oranges

3 qt. water

Directions

1. Combine and chill at least 2 hours.

Muscle Revival

Drink this watermelon infused water before exercise to reduce heart rate and prevent muscle soreness the day after.

Ingredients

1/2 cup seedless, cubed watermelon,

1 Tbsp fresh, chopped mint

Directions

1. Add the watermelon and mint to a 20-oz. bottle.

2. Fill the bottle with water. For maximum flavor, chill overnight.

No-More-Nausea Ginger Ale

Ingredients

Ginger is a natural remedy for nausea. It is also safe.

6 cups of water

Juice from 2 lemons

1 ginger root, washed & peeled

Directions

1. Place the water in a medium-size pan. Add the juice from the lemons and add the ginger root.

2. Heat this mixture on high heat until it boils. Cover saucepan and lower the heat.

3. Simmer for 10 to 15 minutes. Drink it hot, poured over ice or chilled.

Relaxation Sage Waters

Ingredients

Sage is renowned for its comforting and relaxing effect.

1/4cup crushed pineapple

1/4cup crushed raspberries

2 fresh sage leaves

16 oz. water

Directions

1. Add fruits and vegetables to water. Refrigerate for at least 2hrs.

2. If in hurry, place in the freezer for 10 minutes. Stir thoroughly then sip.

No-More-Nausea Sweet Ginger Ale

Ingredients

6 cups of water

Juice from 1 lemon

Juice from 1 orange

1 ginger root, washed & peeled

Directions

1. Place the water in a medium-size pan. Add the juice from the lemons, orange and then add ginger root.

2. Heat this mixture on high heat until it boils. Cover saucepan and lower the heat.

3. Simmer for 10 to 15 minutes. Drink it hot, poured over ice or chilled.

Beautiful Skin Vitamin Water

Maintain a beautiful skin by taking this regularly. It is packed full of vitamins and also has inflammatory ingredients that will benefit you.

Ingredients

2 cups cubed watermelon

1 cup strawberries

2 sprigs fresh rosemary

Filtered water

Dash of salt

Directions

1. Muddle the rosemary and strawberries in a bowl.

2. Add together with the watermelon to a pitcher.

3. Pour water over it, stir gently and chill for 4 hours.

FRUIT INFUSED WATER RECIPES FOR DETOX

Great Year Detox Mix

Burn fat, boost your metabolism and flush out nasty toxins.

Ingredients

1 gallon pitcher water

3 raspberries

Grapefruit, sliced

Cucumber, sliced

Pears, sliced

1 sprig of fresh mint

Directions

1. Add all the ingredients together.

2. Chill for a few hours to combine the flavors. Enjoy!

Grapefruit Rosemary Infusion

Ingredients

½ grapefruit

Several rosemary sprigs

Directions

1. Add to a pitcher. Fill with water.

2. Leave overnight and drink the next day.

Blood Orange & Pineapple Mint

Ingredients

1 handful of pineapple mint

1 blood orange, sliced

1 cup sliced strawberries

2 quarts water

Directions:

1. In a 2 quart pitcher, add all the ingredients together.

2. Refrigerate overnight. Enjoy the next day.

Kiwi Strawberry Water

Kiwi contains vitamins A and E which helps to remove free radicals from the body. They also help to eradicate toxins from the colon. Strawberries help in fighting carcinogens.

Ingredients

2 strawberries, chopped

2 kiwis, chopped

2 liters of water

Directions

1. Add the strawberries and kiwis to water and let it sit refrigerated for a few hours.

2. Enjoy your drink

No- Calorie Apple Cinnamon

This delicious water contains no calories; but that is not all. It helps to eliminate harmful toxins from your body while boosting your metabolism and keeping you in great shape!

Ingredients

1 apple, thinly sliced

1 cinnamon stick

Directions

1. Add the apple and cinnamon to water.

2. Fill with ice or refrigerate.

Pomegranate & Blueberry Infused Water
Ingredients:

1/2 cup pomegranate seeds

1 pint blueberries, fresh

2 quarts water

Directions:

1. Add the blueberries and pomegranate seeds to a 2 quart pitcher.

2. Fill with water and store in the fridge for 2-4 hours.

2–In-1 Detox Water

This recipe flushes out nasty toxins and aids weight loss. Apple cider vinegar is extremely beneficial to the body, cinnamon helps to curb appetite. Apples are great fibers and lemons have cleansing properties.

Ingredients

1 tablespoon fresh lemon juice

½ medium apple, sliced

1 teaspoon ground cinnamon

2 tablespoons apple cider vinegar

12 ounces filtered water

Sweetener, optional

Directions

1. Add all the ingredients, except the apples to a blender and blend 10-15 seconds.

2. Now add the apples and drink.

Combo Detox Water

The lemon in this fruit infused recipe helps to boost your immune system and clean out harmful toxins. Cucumber helps you to remain hydrated and it is also anti–inflammatory as well. Mint aids in digestion.

Ingredients

10-12 mint leaves

1 medium cucumber, sliced

1 lemon, sliced

8 cups of water

Directions

1. Add all the ingredients to a large pitcher, mixing thoroughly.

2. Refrigerate overnight and enjoy this tasty detox drink the following day.

Aloe Gel Water

Taking aloe internally can help with digestion and circulation, energy increase as well as fatigue elimination.

Ingredients

2 tablespoons aloe gel from aloe leaf

2 tablespoon lemon juice

1 cup water

Directions

1. To get the aloe gel, split the leaf down at the centre and take out the gel.

2. Next, mix the gel with the lemon and water in the blender and process for 1-2 minutes.

Lemon And Ginger Infusion

Adding ginger to your water is great for detox. As a natural pain reliever, you are pain-free all through the day. The lemon juice added works by helping to release nasty toxins so that they will flush out better.

Ingredients

12 oz of water

Juice of ½ of a lemon

½ inch fresh ginger root knob, grated

Directions

1. Add the lemon juice to the water and add the grated ginger.

2. This is best taken in the morning.

Flavorful Pineapple And Ginger

Ingredients:

1 cup of fresh pineapple pieces

1-inch piece ginger, sliced thinly

2 quarts water

Directions:

1. Add the ginger and pineapple to a 2 quarts pitcher.

2. Pour water over it and place in a refrigerator for a few hours.

Serve over ice.

Ginger-Kumquat Medley

Ingredients

2 cups of kumquats, sliced with seeds removed

1-inch piece fresh ginger, peeled

3 fresh mint stems

2 quarts water

Ice

Directions:

1. Add the ginger to a large pitcher then muddle it with a wooden spoon.

2. Next, squeeze the mint leaves and add it to the pitcher.

3. Add the kumquats and fill the pitcher up with water.

4. Let it chill for at least one hour to infuse well.

5. Serve with ice.

FRUIT INFUSED WATER RECIPES FOR WEIGHT LOSS

Weight loss & Detox infused Water

Eliminate toxins and fat with this recipe. Cucumbers prevent water retention. Limes and lemons help in flushing out toxins and grapefruits help in burning fat.

Ingredients

½ medium grapefruit, sliced

½ a cucumber, sliced

½ lemon, sliced

½ lime, sliced

½ gallon of spring water

2 mint leaves

Directions

1. Add the ingredients together and refrigerate for 4-6 hours.

2. Serve and drink daily for optimal results.

Cranberry Lemon Infusion

Ingredients:

1 cup of fresh cranberries

1 lemon, sliced

1 handful mint

2 quarts of water

Directions:

1. Use a wooden spoon to muddle the cranberries and then slice the mint and lemon.

2. Place in a jar and fill it with water

3. Refrigerate for about two hours.

Citrus Relish

Ingredients:

1 lime, sliced

1 orange, sliced

2 quarts water

Directions:

1. Fill a 2 quarts pitcher with water.

2. To it, add the lime and orange. (To release more juice, squeeze some of the slices).

3. Stir and chill for at least 2hour before drinking.

Mango- Orange Mix

Ingredients

2 oranges, quartered

2 mangoes, ripe & thinly sliced

2 quarts water

Ice

Directions:

1. Add all the ingredients together in a 2 quart jar.

2. Refrigerate 2 hours and enjoy.

Orange Cranberry Water

This infused water is calorie free and refreshing for the hot weather.

Ingredients

1 cup of fresh cranberries

1 orange

1 small handful sage

2 quarts water

Directions:

1. Smash the cranberries and slice the orange thinly.

2. Add this to the pitcher and fill with water.

3. Refrigerate for two hours.

Cantaloupe And Strawberry Delight

Ingredients

1 pint strawberries, hulled &quartered

1 cup cantaloupe cubes

2 quarts water

Directions:

1. Combine all the ingredients in a pitcher.

2. Let it chill for several hours.

3. Serve the chilled drink with ice

Mixed Melon Infused Water

With leftover melons, you can make this refreshing infusion at any time.

Ingredients:

1 cup of honeydew pieces

1 cup cantaloupe pieces

1 cup watermelon pieces

2 quarts of water

Directions:

1. Add together all ingredients. (Use a jar or pitcher).

2. Pour water to it then refrigerate two hours.

END

www.ingramcontent.com/pod-product-compliance
Lightning Source LLC
Chambersburg PA
CBHW050515290526
45786CB00007B/2576